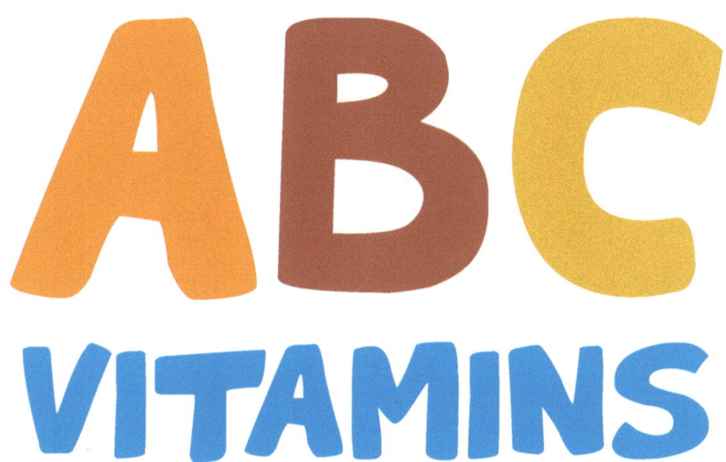

By Brianna Huff

To my nieces, Bailey, Julia, and Sophie
for reminding me to keep my imagination alive.

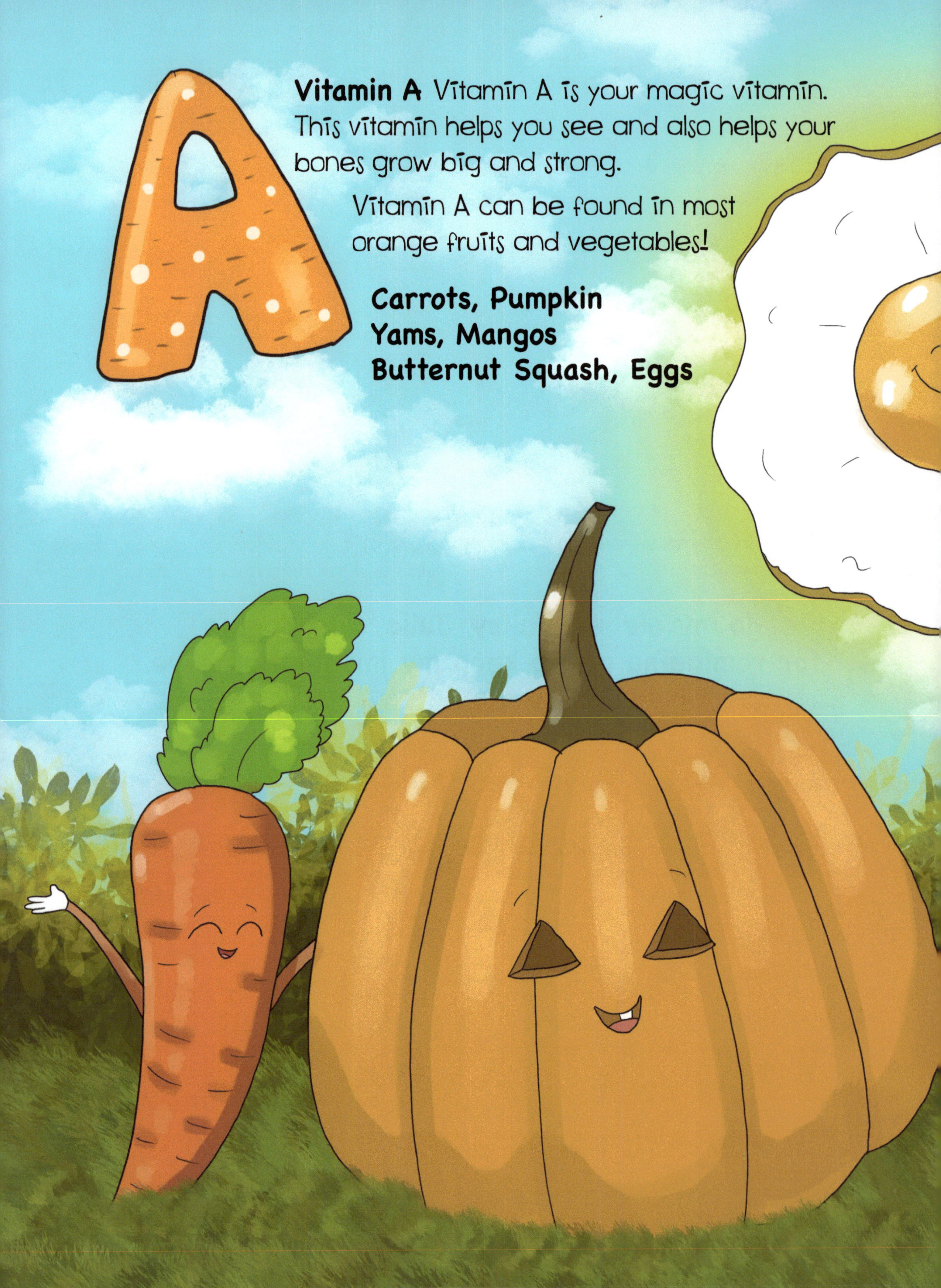

Vitamin A Vitamin A is your magic vitamin. This vitamin helps you see and also helps your bones grow big and strong.
Vitamin A can be found in most orange fruits and vegetables!
Carrots, Pumpkin
Yams, Mangos
Butternut Squash, Eggs

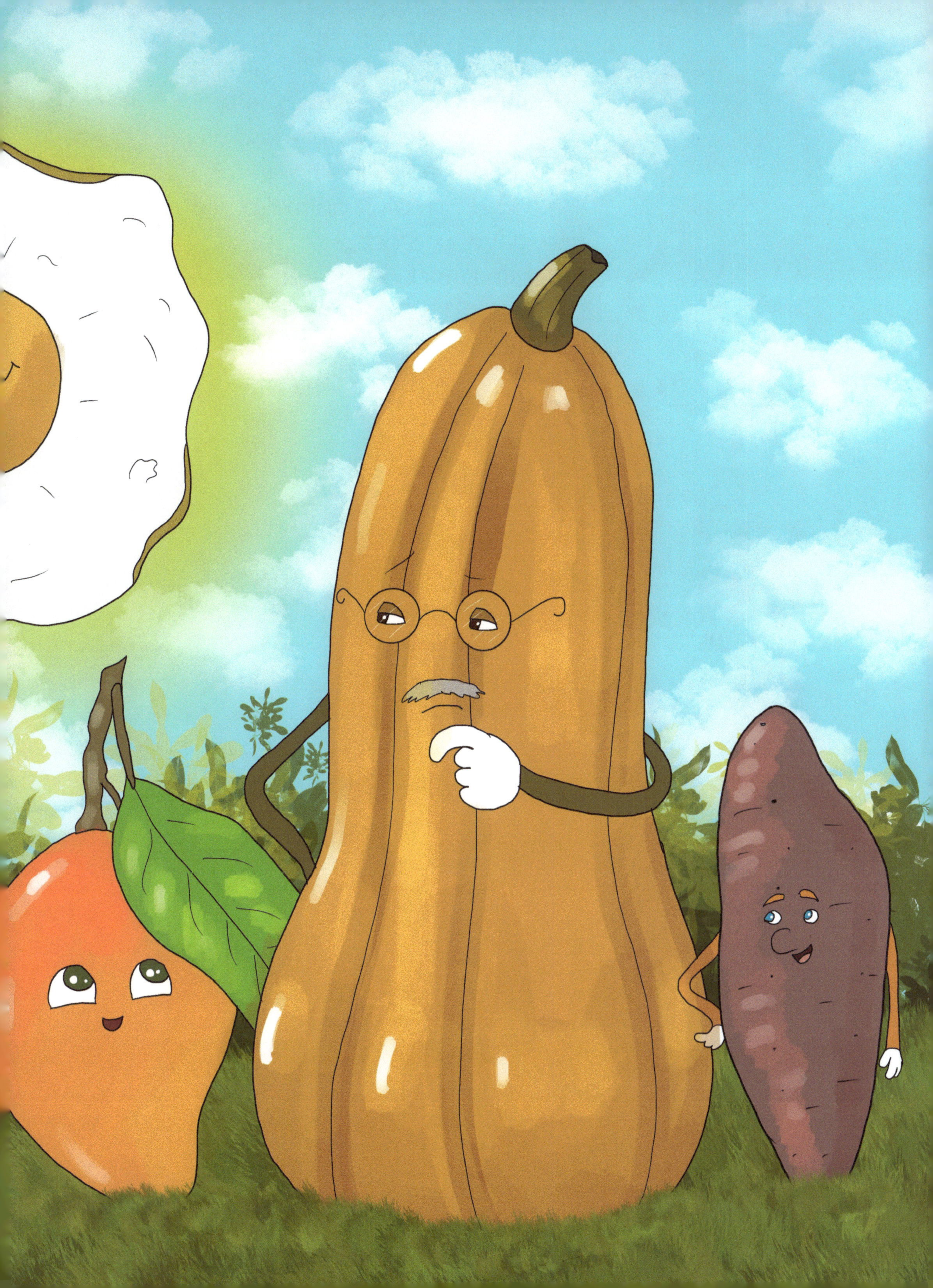

B

Vitamin B is your energy vitamin. Vitamin B keeps your heart healthy and without it, you would be tired all the time. This vitamin can be found in mainly animal-based foods like meat, fish, and eggs.

Vitamin B includes B1, B2, B3, B5, B6, and B12.

Vitamin B1 (Thiamin)

Vitamin B1 helps the body's cells change carbs into energy. The main job of carbs is to give you energy.

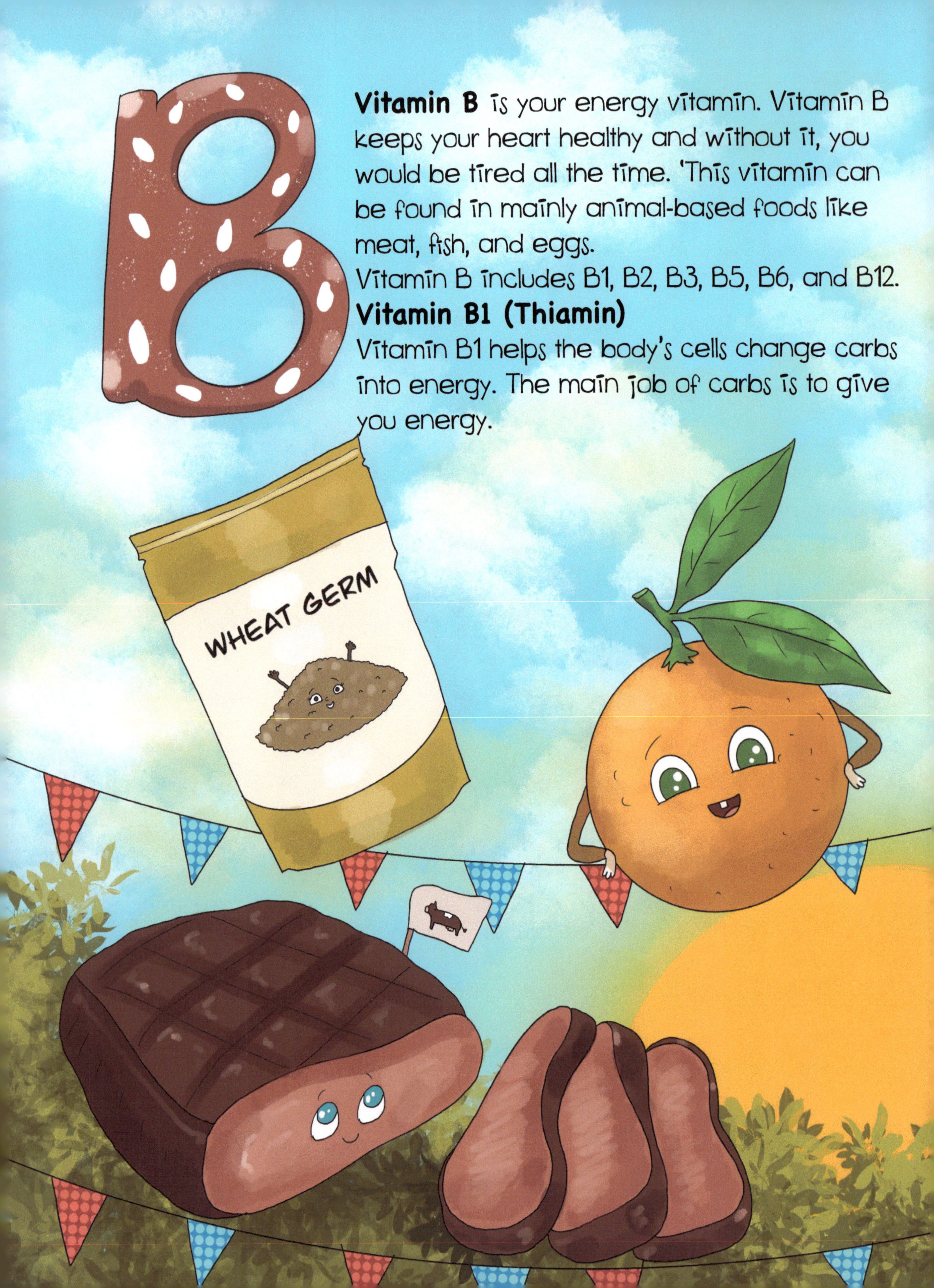

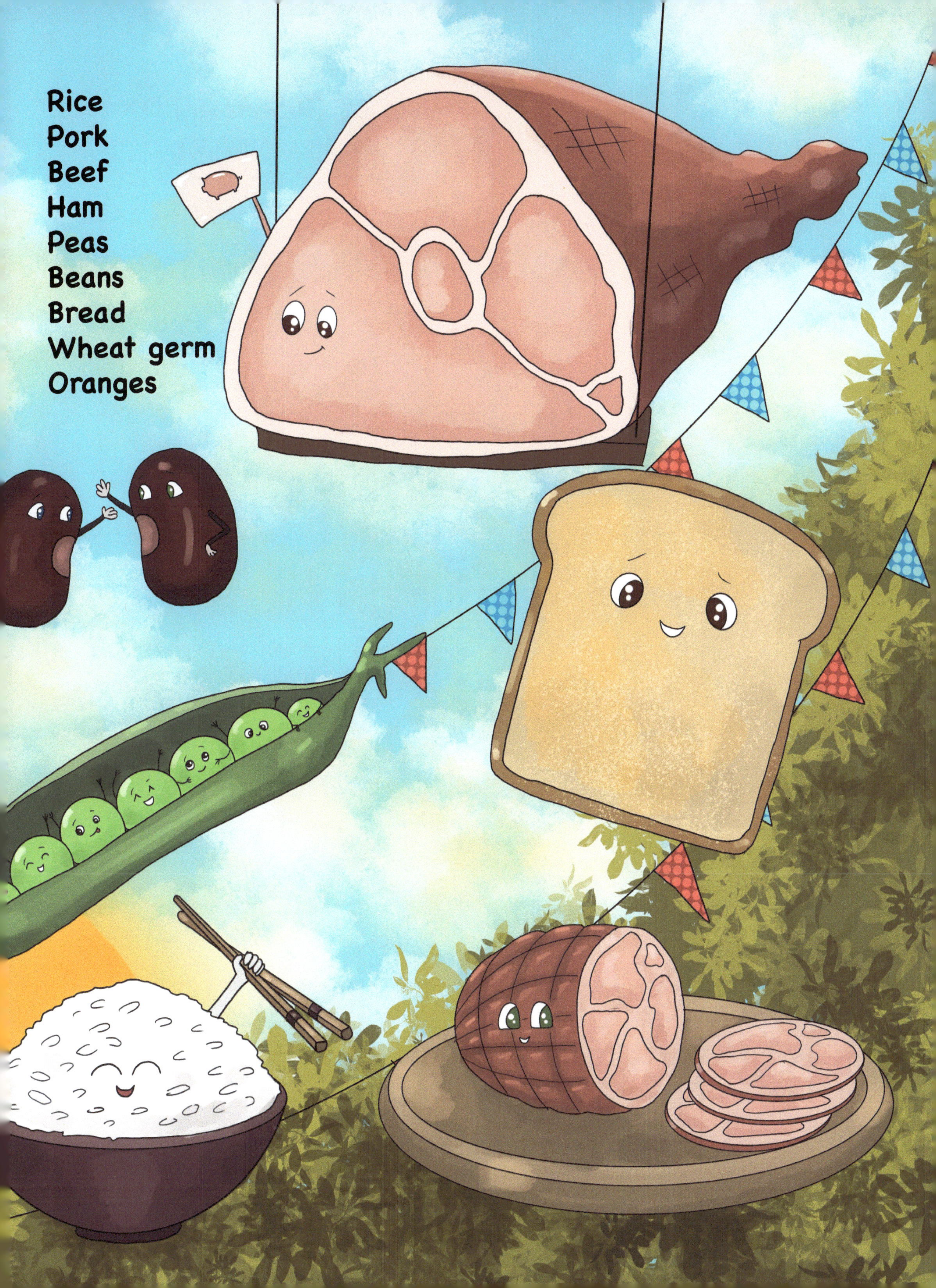

Rice
Pork
Beef
Ham
Peas
Beans
Bread
Wheat germ
Oranges

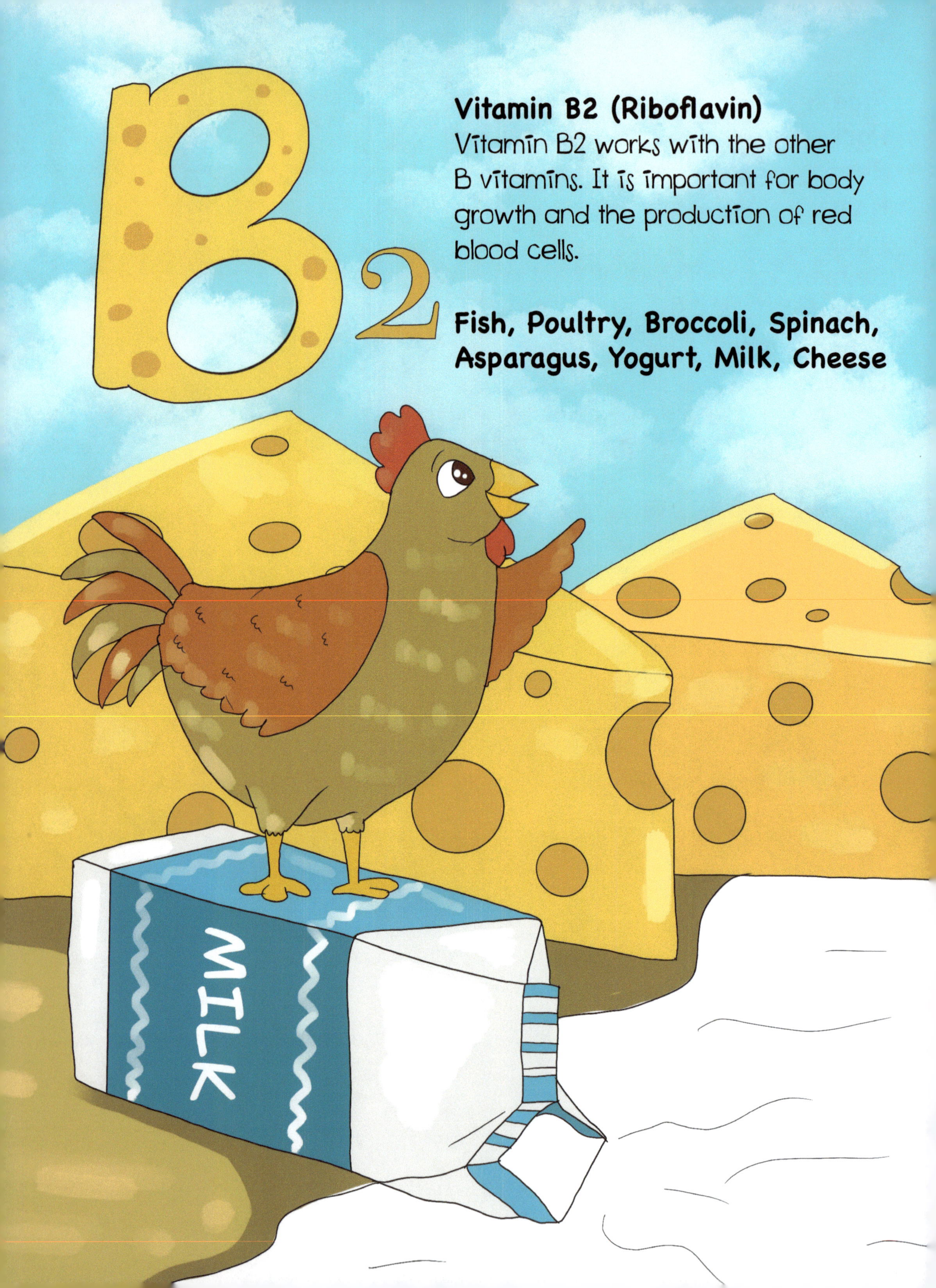

Vitamin B2 (Riboflavin)
Vitamin B2 works with the other B vitamins. It is important for body growth and the production of red blood cells.

Fish, Poultry, Broccoli, Spinach, Asparagus, Yogurt, Milk, Cheese

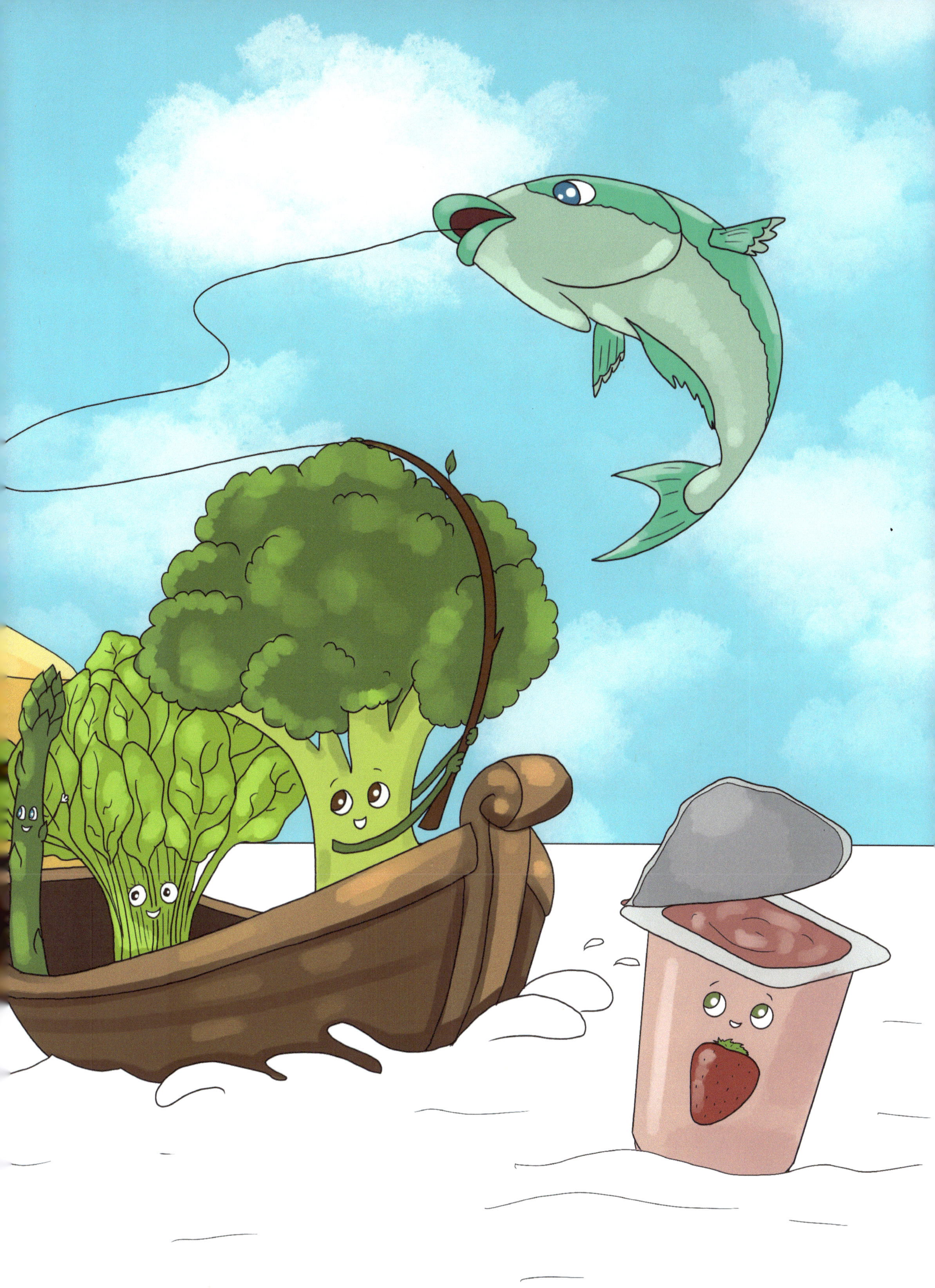

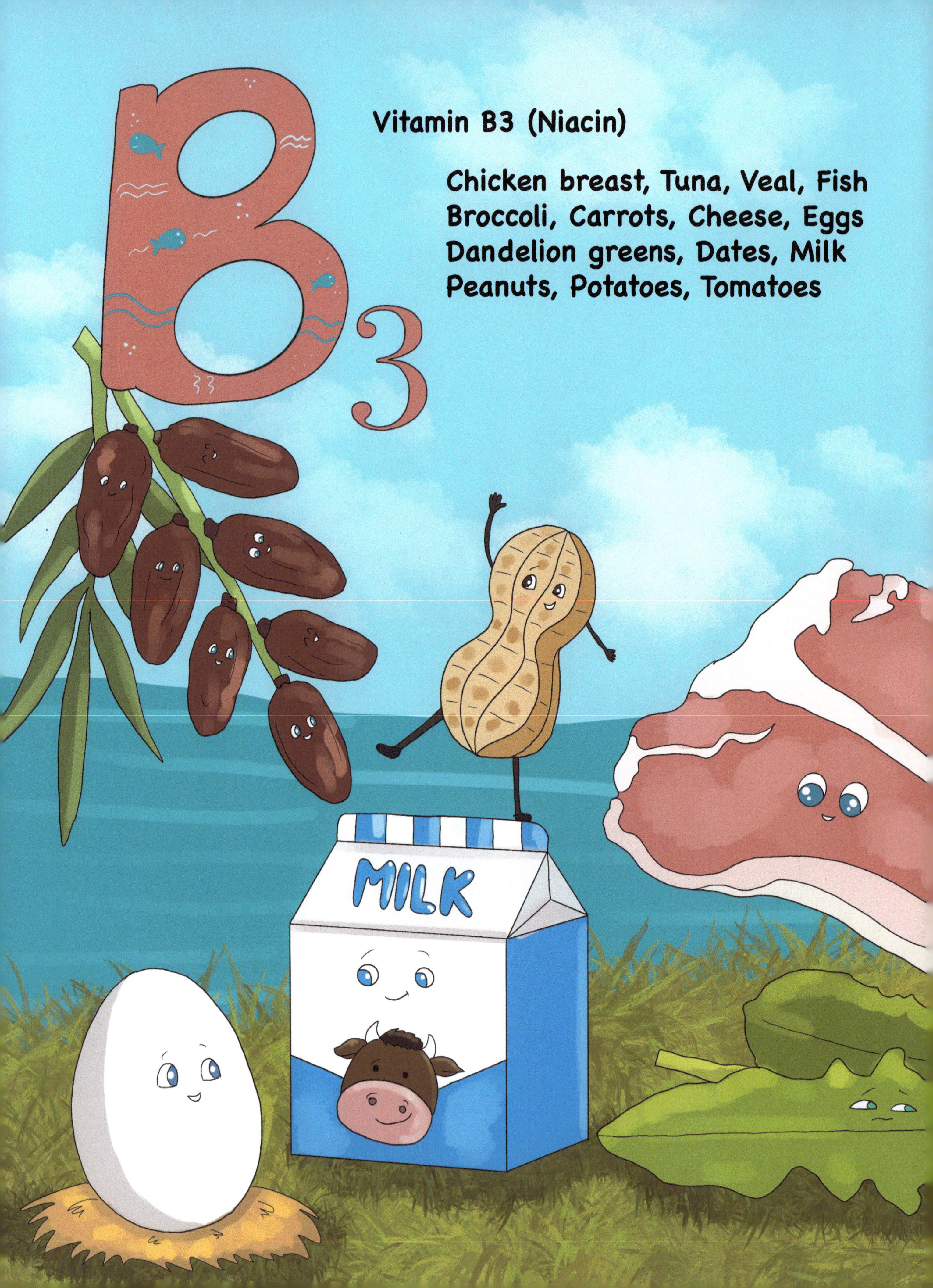

B3

Vitamin B3 (Niacin)

Chicken breast, Tuna, Veal, Fish
Broccoli, Carrots, Cheese, Eggs
Dandelion greens, Dates, Milk
Peanuts, Potatoes, Tomatoes

MILK

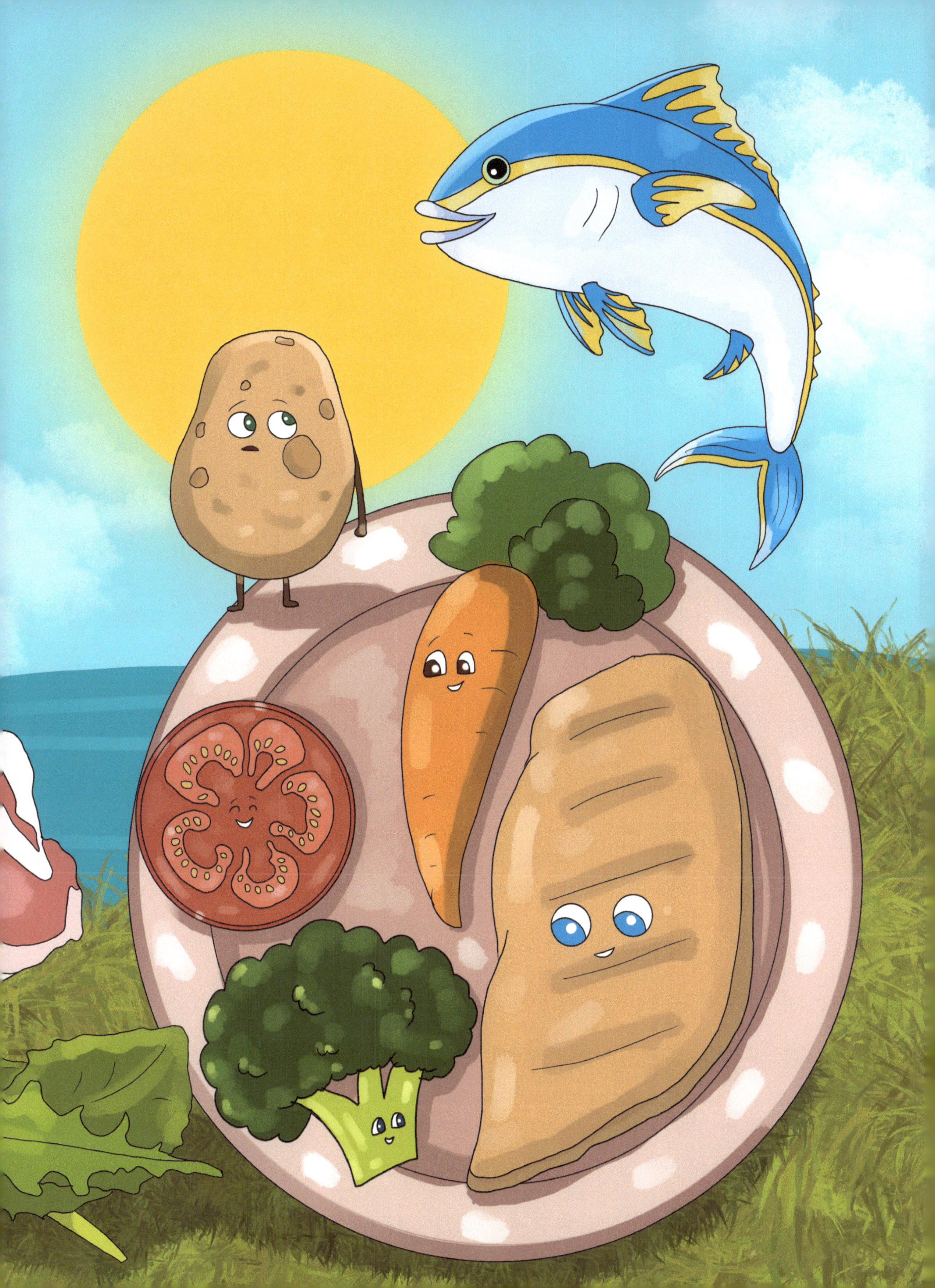

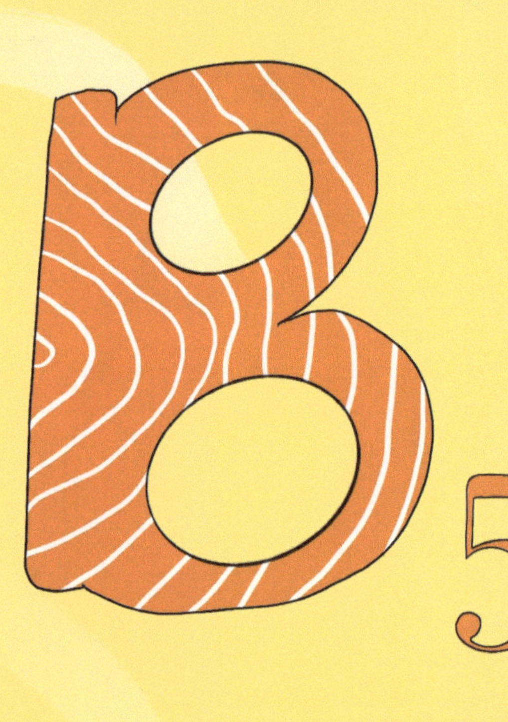

Vitamin B5 (Pantothenic Acid)

Vitamin B5 helps with getting energy from our foods and is good for our skin.

Whole grains, Mushrooms
Salmon, Vegetables, Legumes
Saltwater Fish

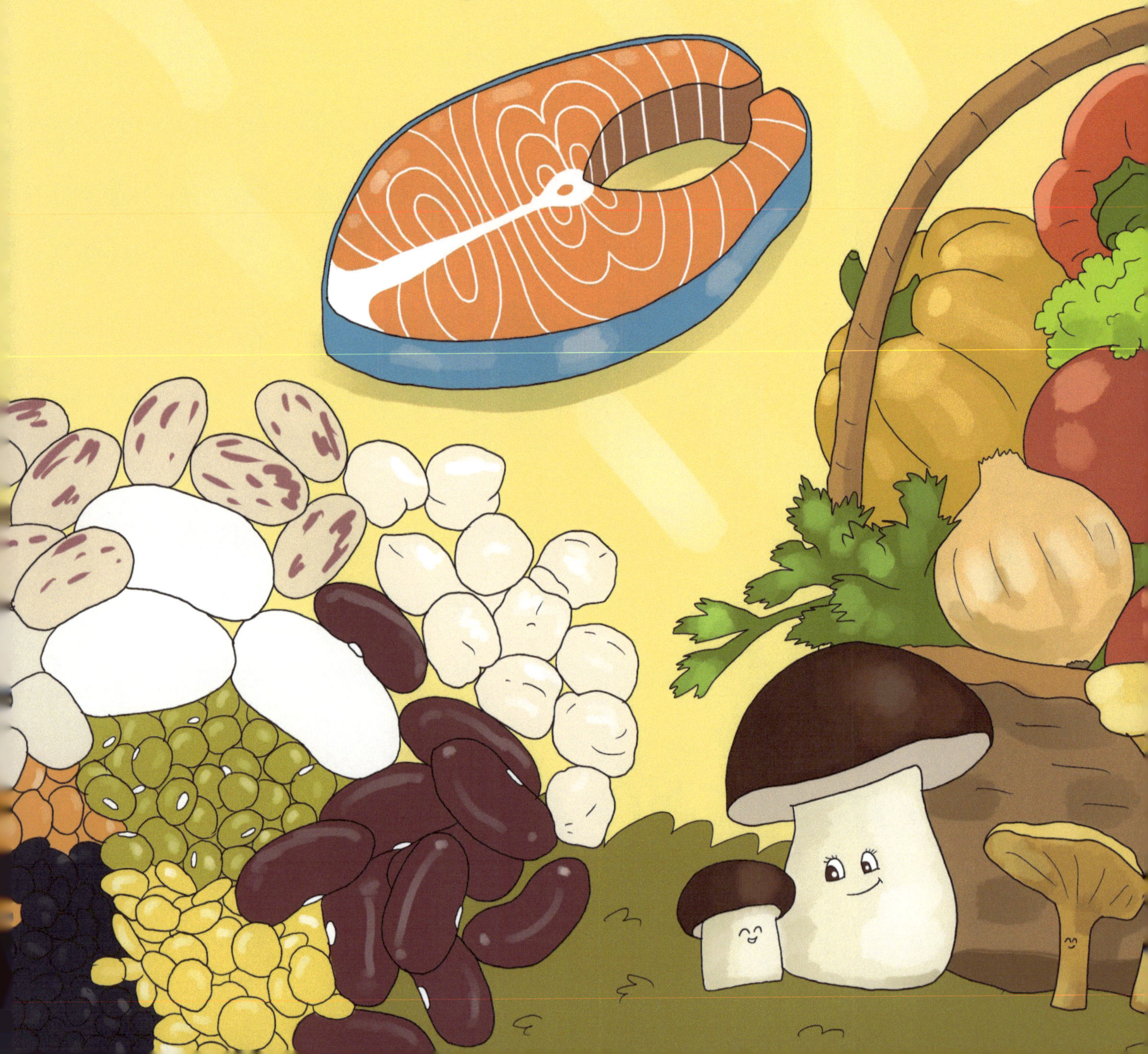

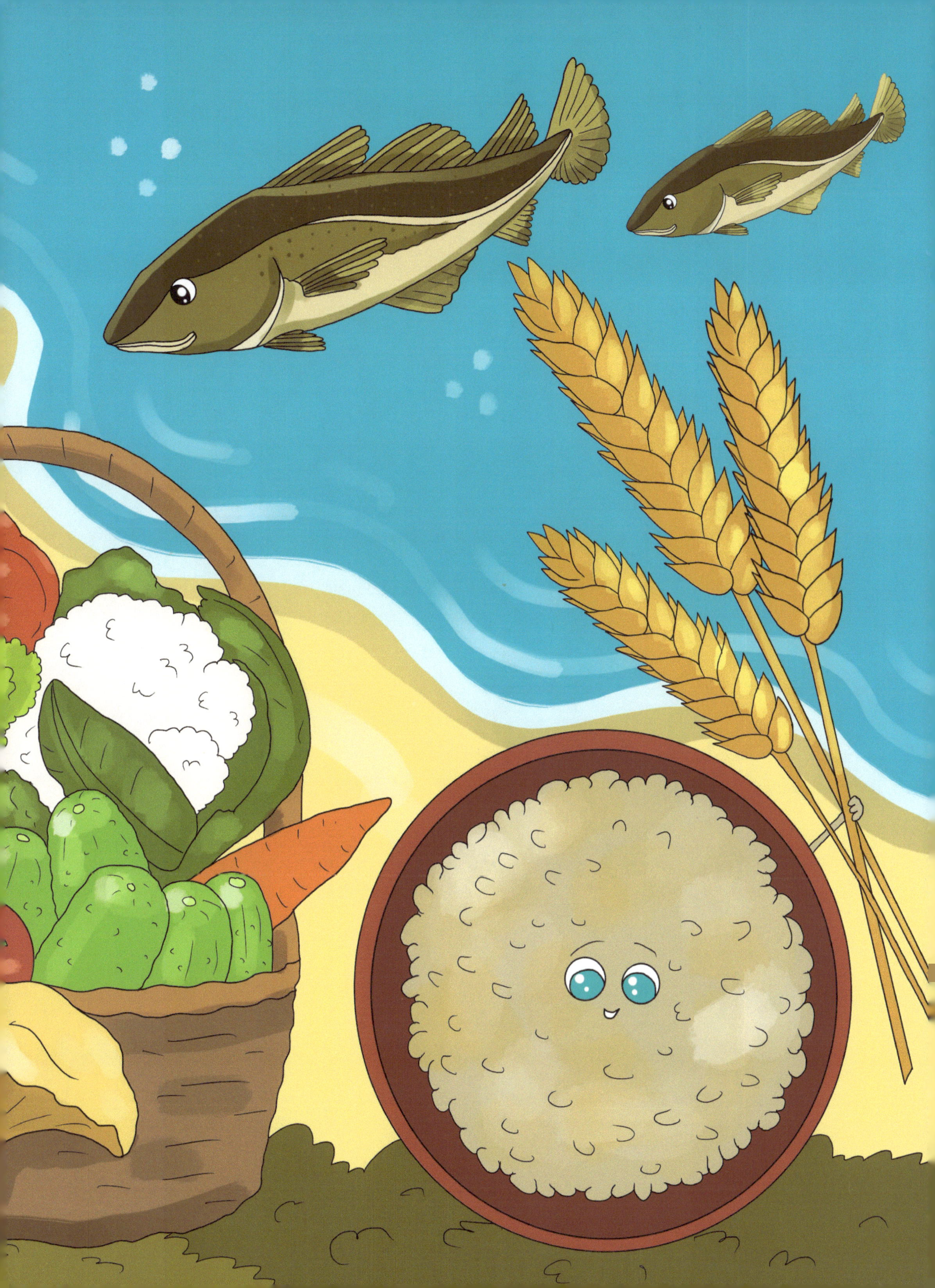

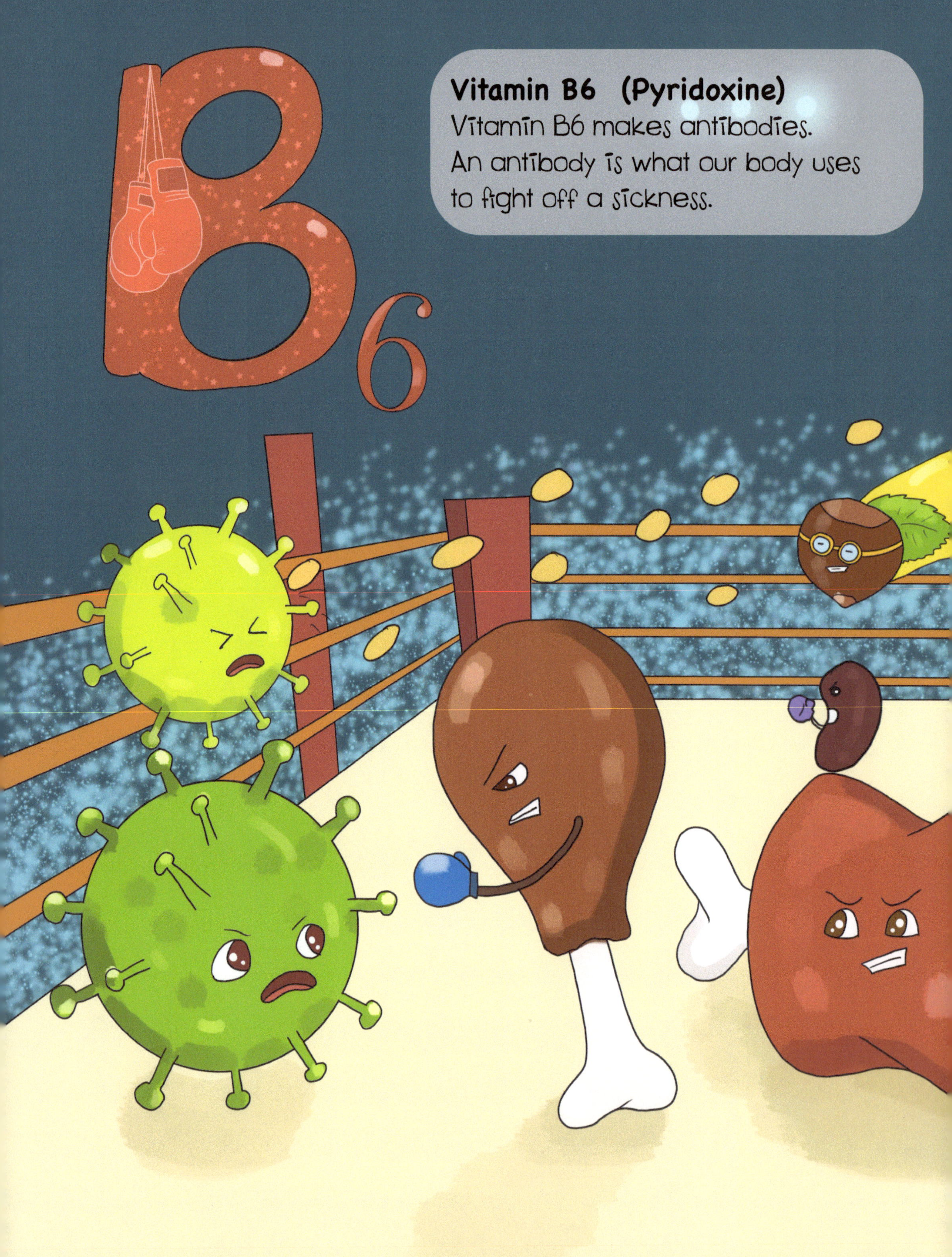
B6
Vitamin B6 (Pyridoxine)
Vitamin B6 makes antibodies.
An antibody is what our body uses
to fight off a sickness.

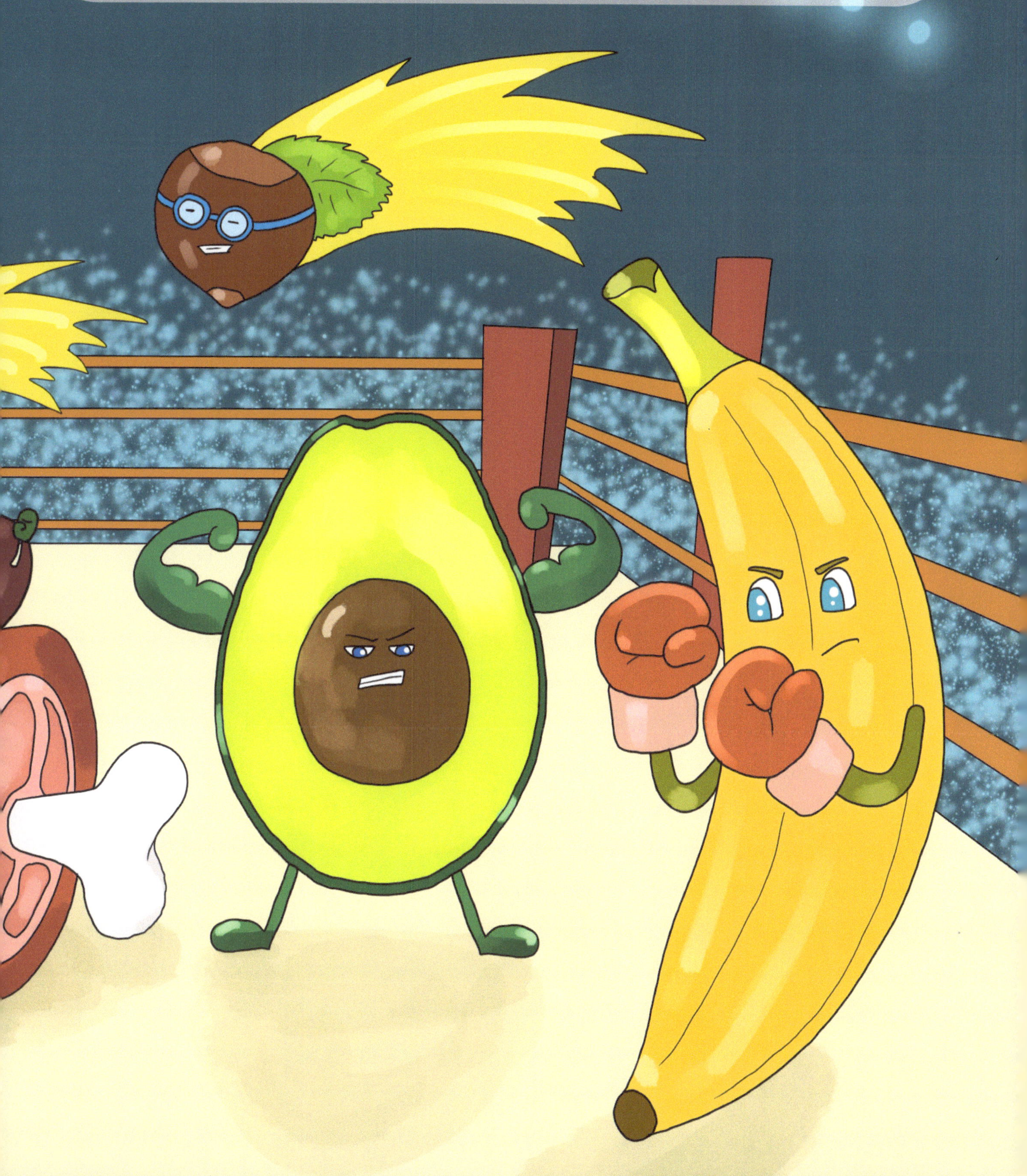
Avocado, Banana, Legumes (dried beans), Meat, Nuts
Poultry, Whole grains (milling and processing removes
a lot of this vitamin)

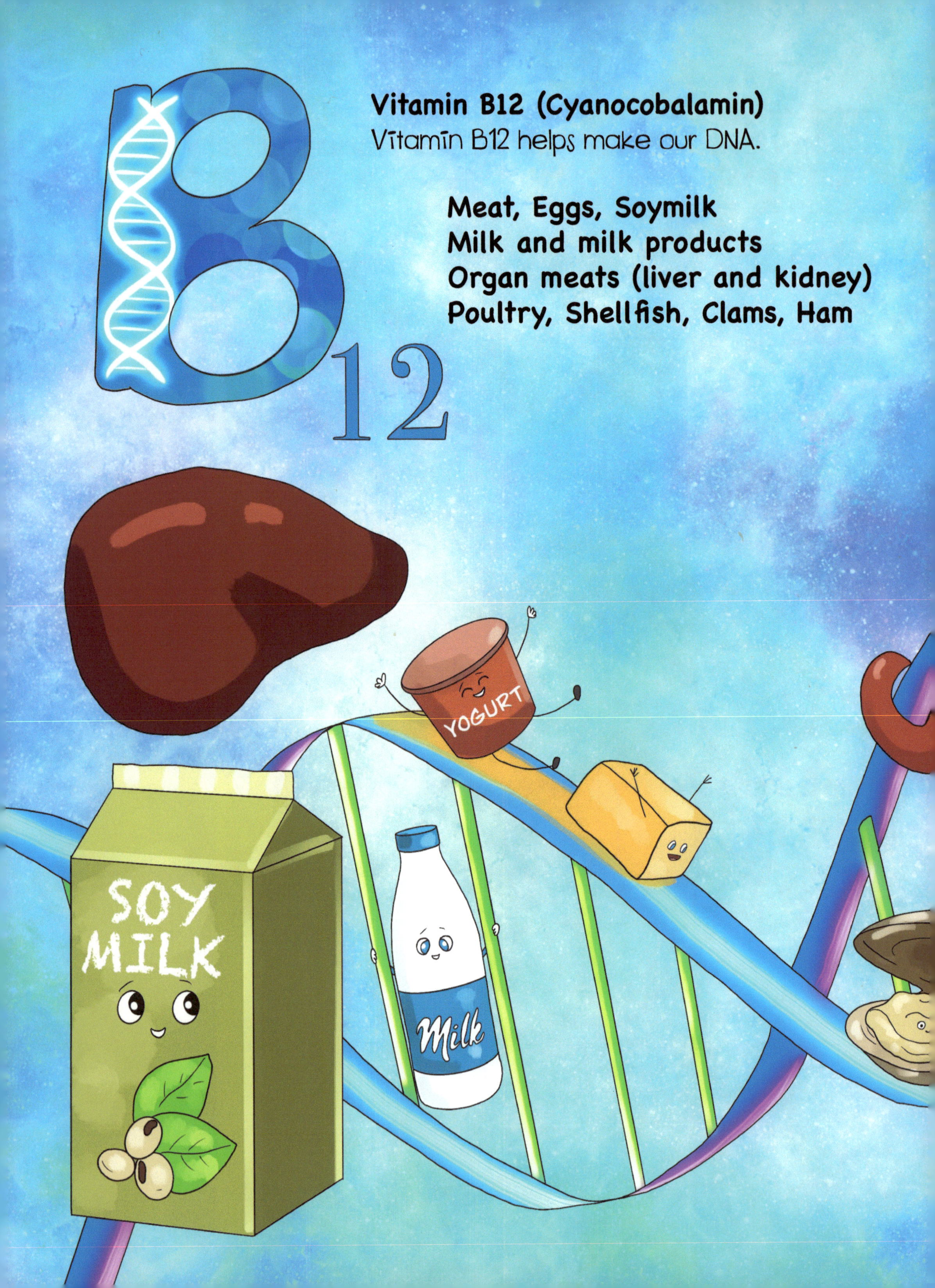

B12

Vitamin B12 (Cyanocobalamin)
Vitamin B12 helps make our DNA.

Meat, Eggs, Soymilk
Milk and milk products
Organ meats (liver and kidney)
Poultry, Shellfish, Clams, Ham

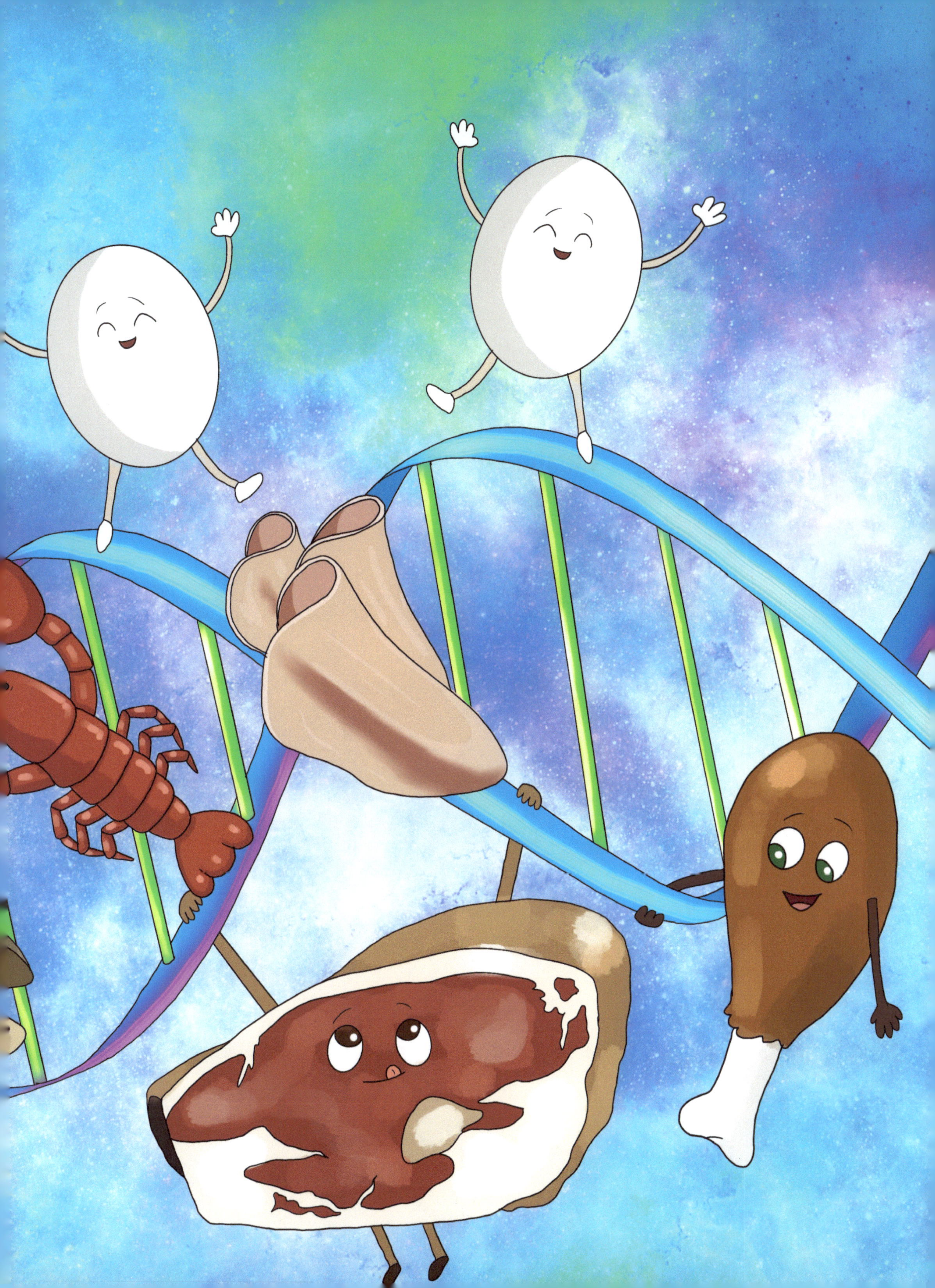

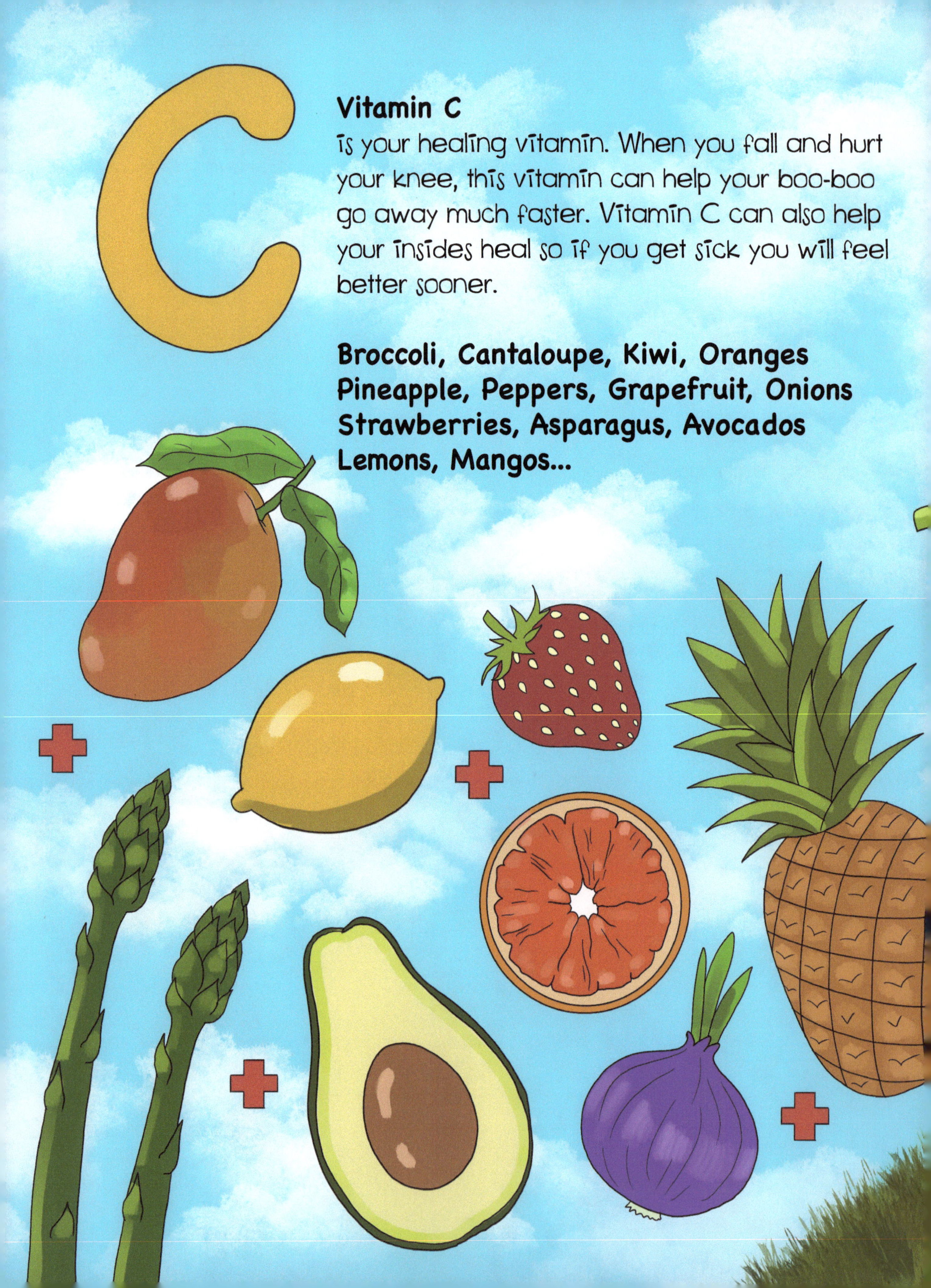

Vitamin C
is your healing vitamin. When you fall and hurt your knee, this vitamin can help your boo-boo go away much faster. Vitamin C can also help your insides heal so if you get sick you will feel better sooner.

Broccoli, Cantaloupe, Kiwi, Oranges
Pineapple, Peppers, Grapefruit, Onions
Strawberries, Asparagus, Avocados
Lemons, Mangos...

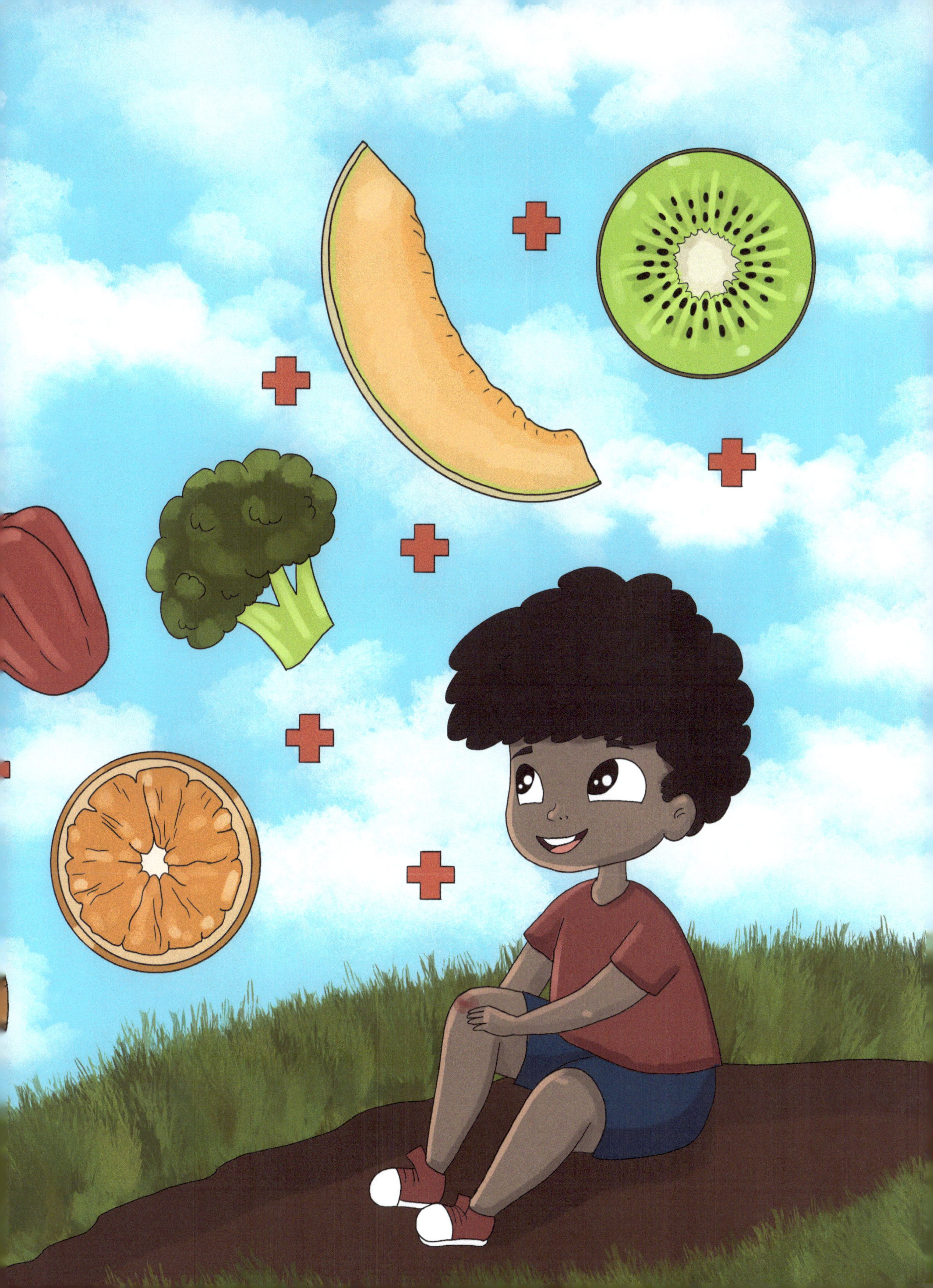

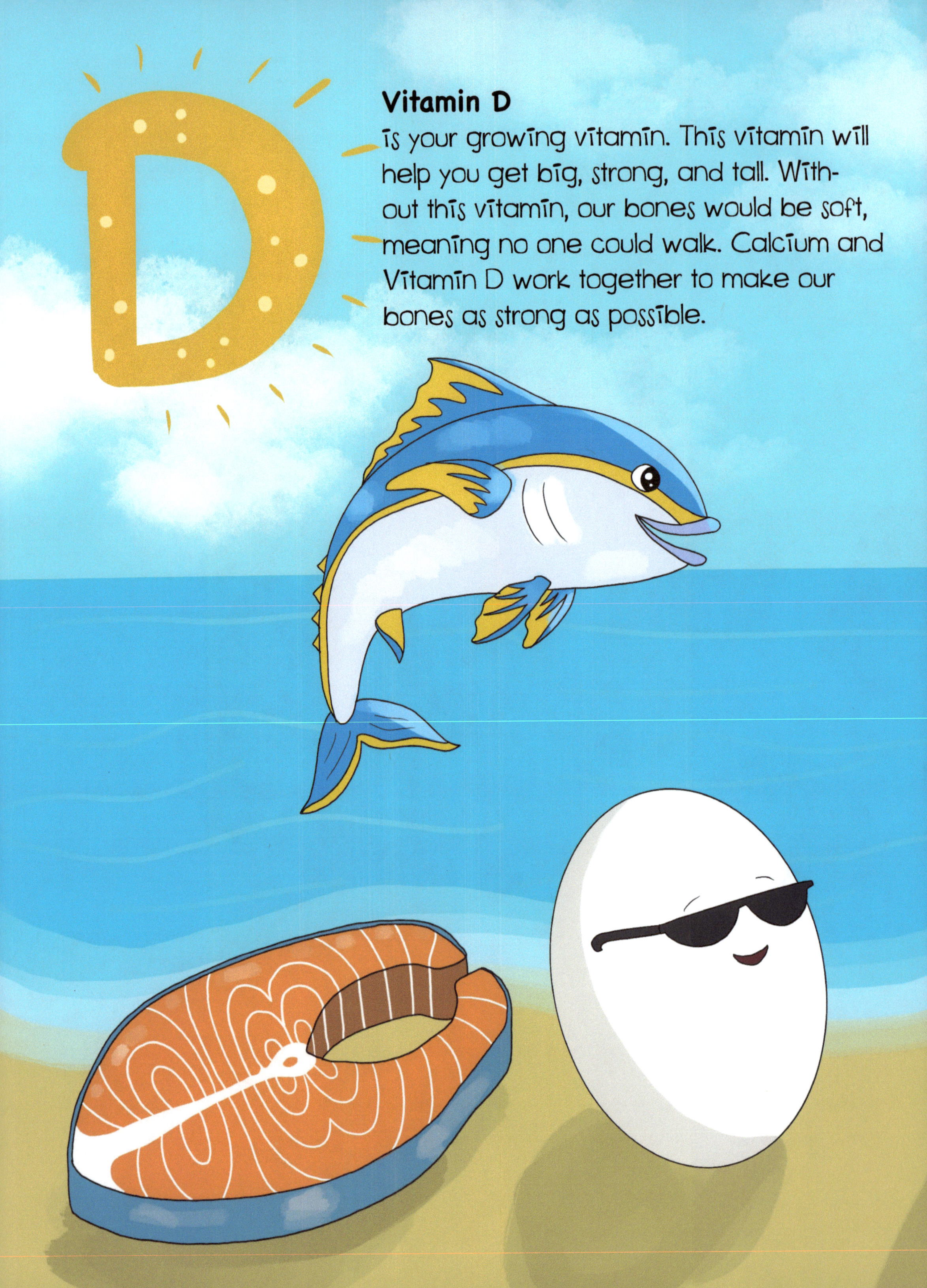

Vitamin D

is your growing vitamin. This vitamin will help you get big, strong, and tall. Without this vitamin, our bones would be soft, meaning no one could walk. Calcium and Vitamin D work together to make our bones as strong as possible.

You can get this vitamin from foods and also from the sun. Playing outside can help you become big and strong.

**Sun exposure
Salmon, Eggs
Mushrooms
Milk, Cereal
Tuna...**

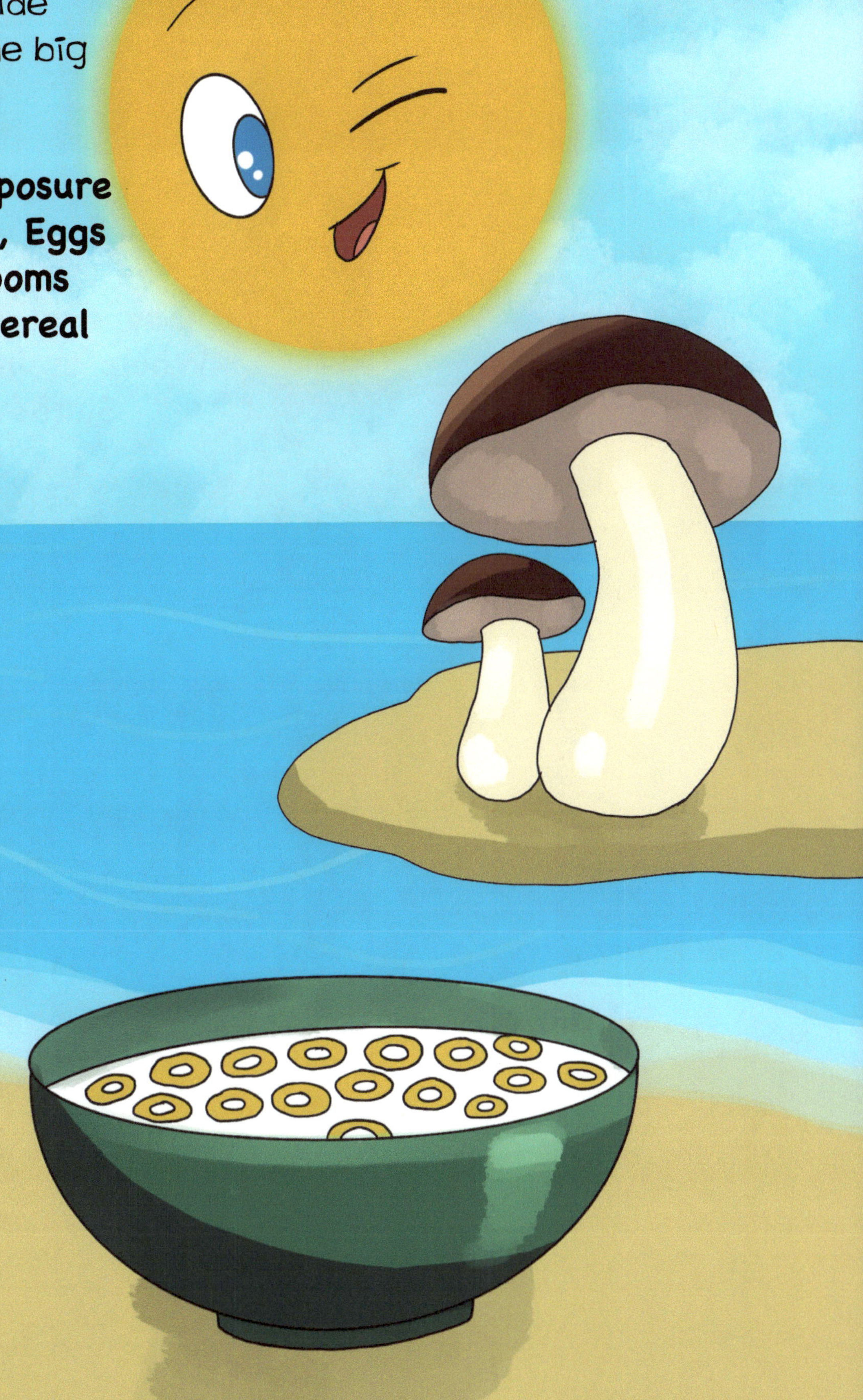

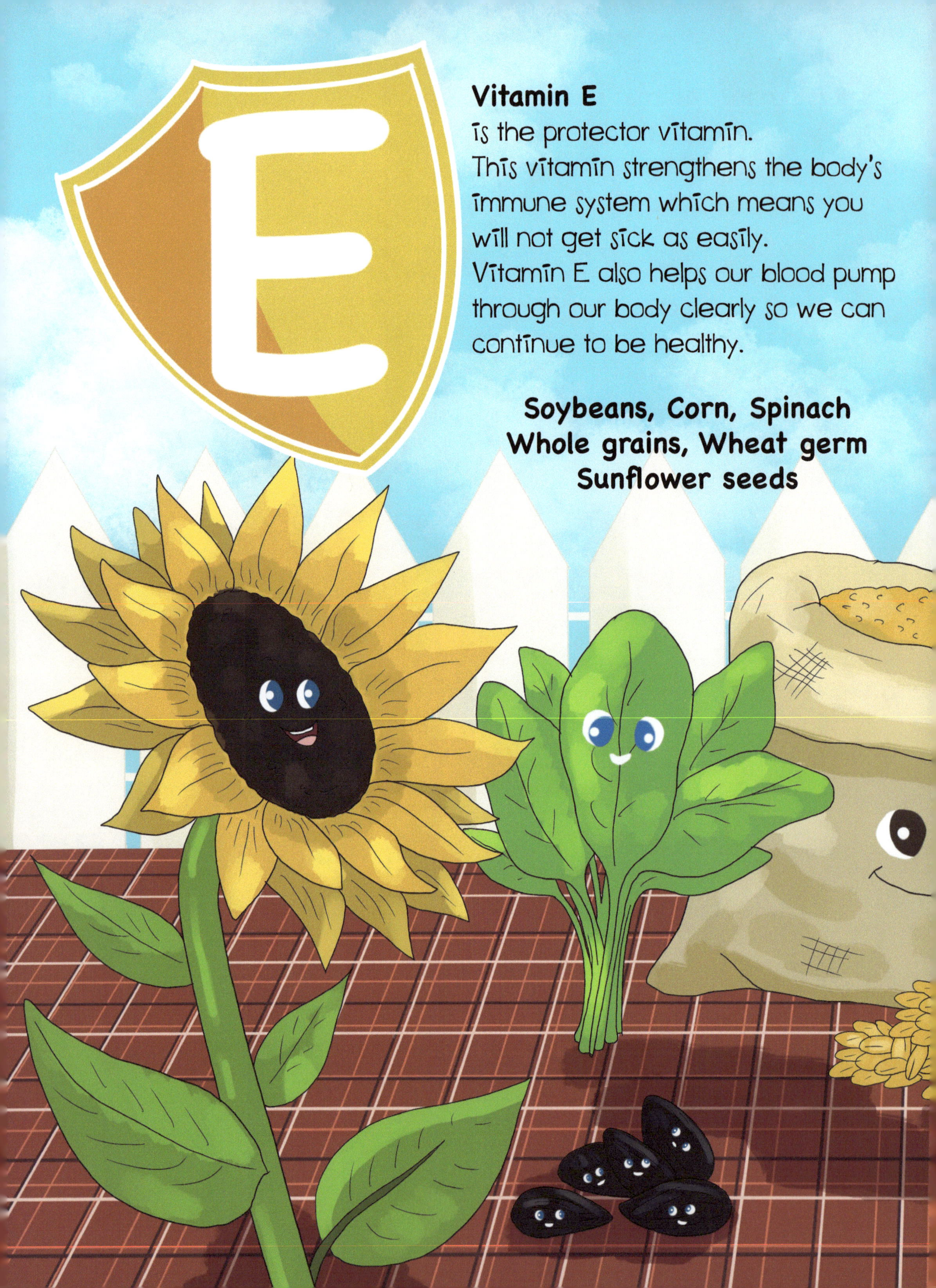

Vitamin E
is the protector vitamin.
This vitamin strengthens the body's
immune system which means you
will not get sick as easily.
Vitamin E also helps our blood pump
through our body clearly so we can
continue to be healthy.

Soybeans, Corn, Spinach
Whole grains, Wheat germ
Sunflower seeds

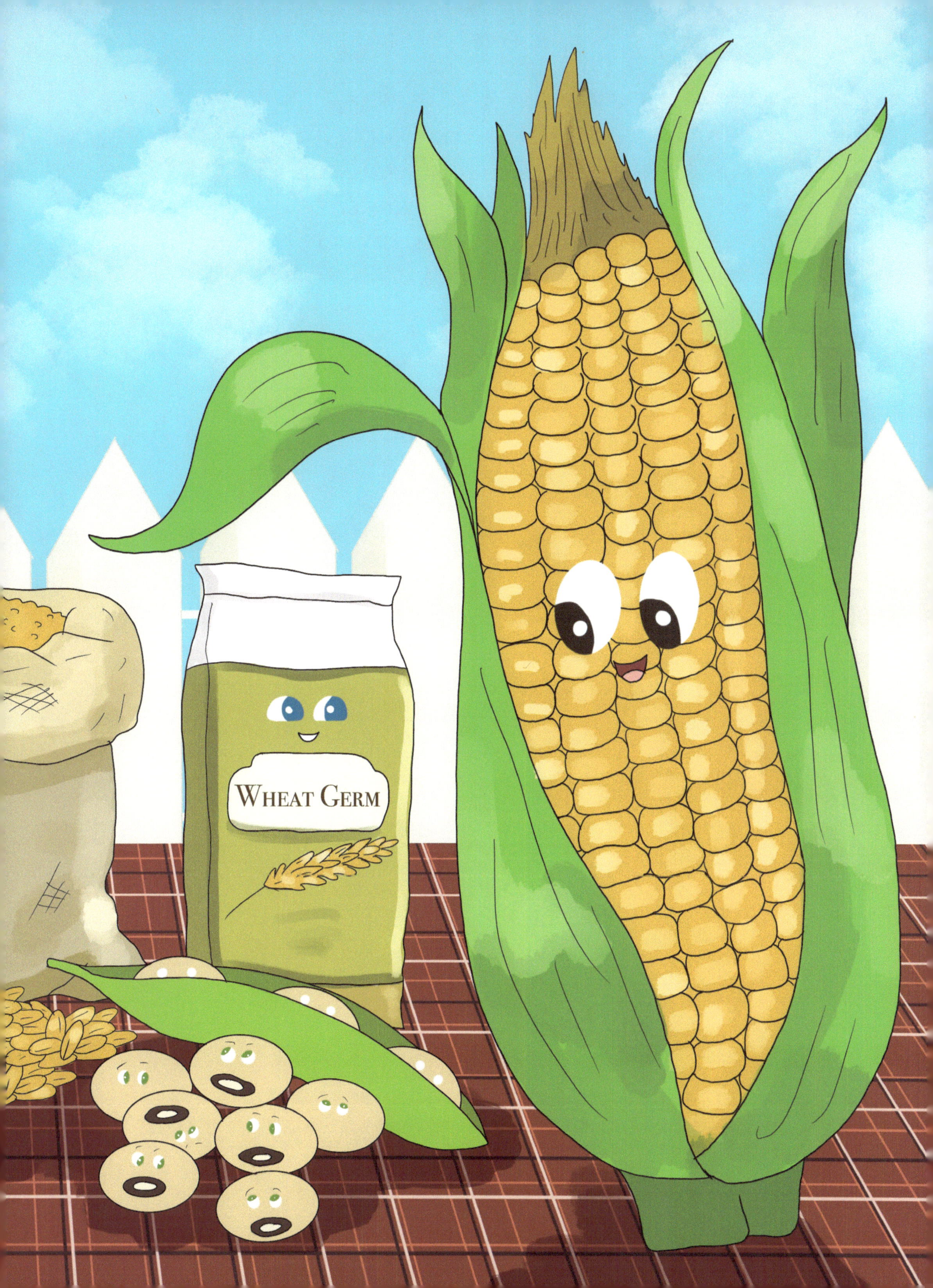
Wheat Germ

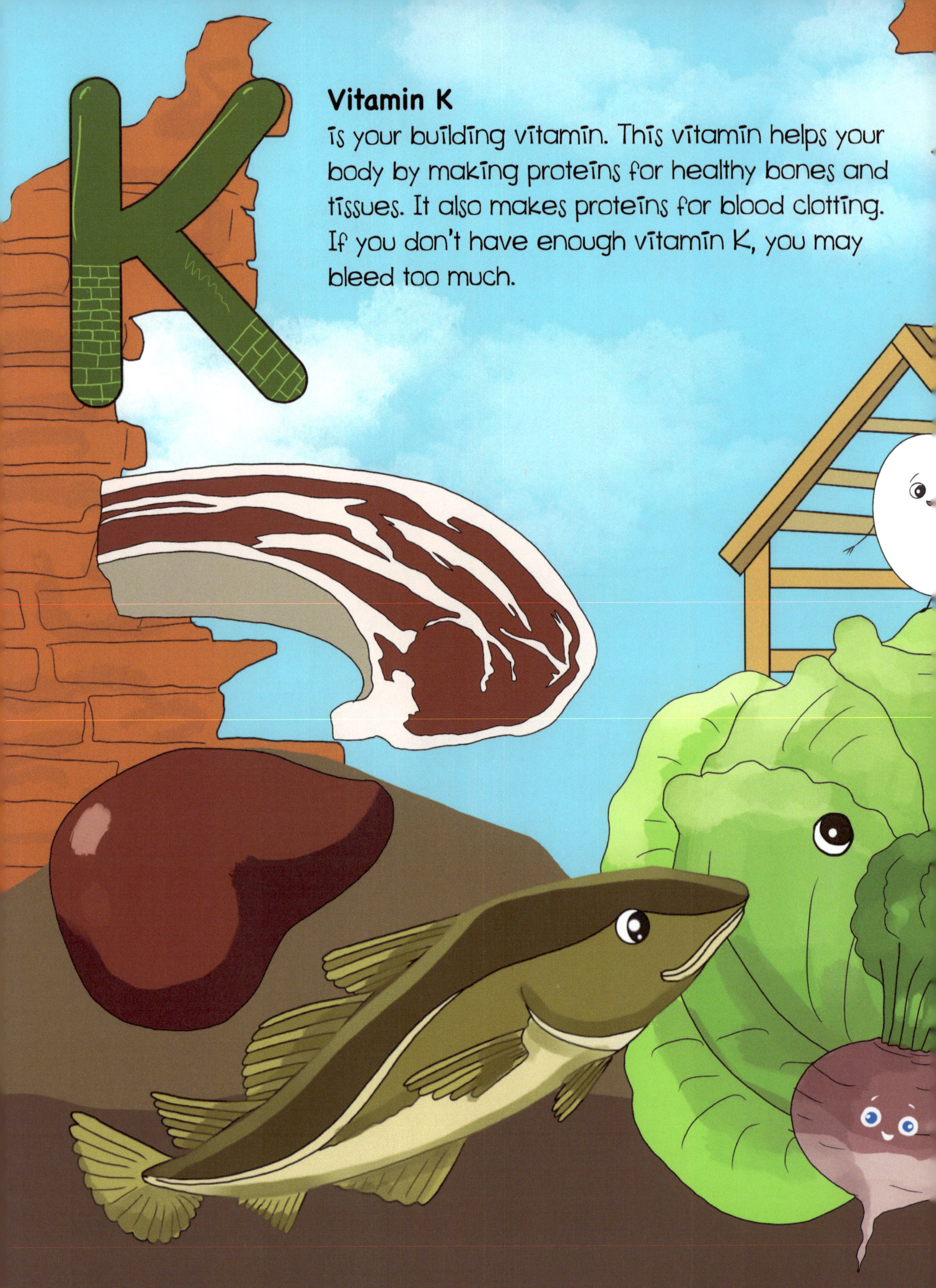

Vitamin K

is your building vitamin. This vitamin helps your body by making proteins for healthy bones and tissues. It also makes proteins for blood clotting. If you don't have enough vitamin K, you may bleed too much.

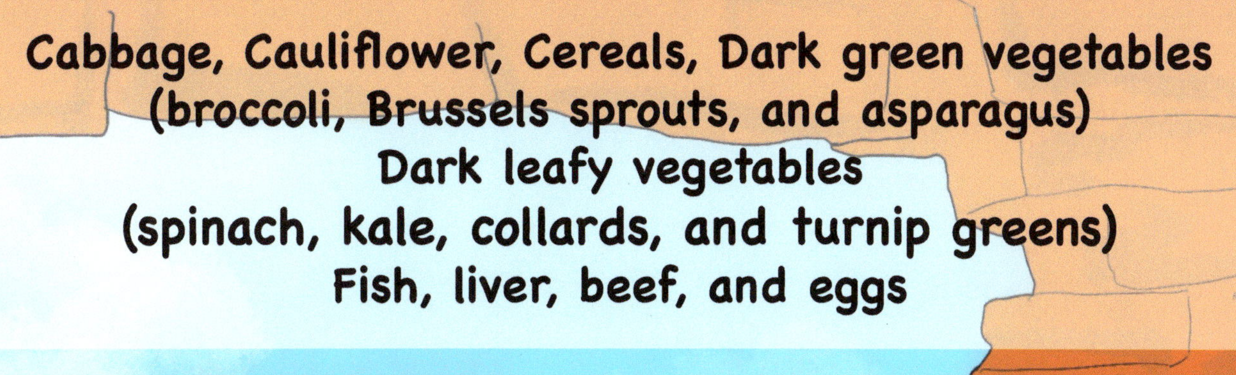

Cabbage, Cauliflower, Cereals, Dark green vegetables
(broccoli, Brussels sprouts, and asparagus)
Dark leafy vegetables
(spinach, kale, collards, and turnip greens)
Fish, liver, beef, and eggs

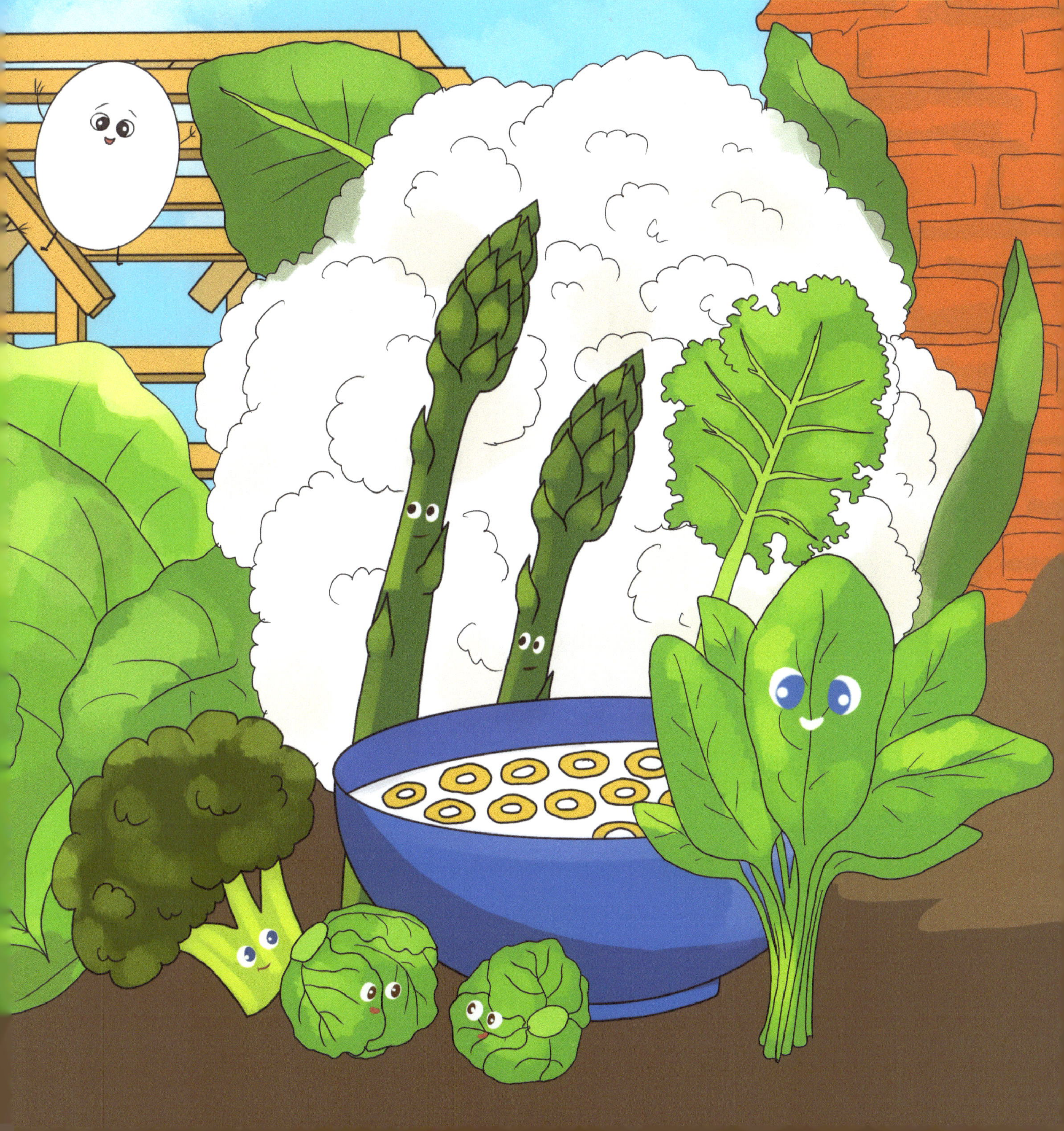

About the author:

Brianna started writing books in 2020
and found a passion for teaching kids.
She is a pre-school teacher while
working on her masters in nutrition.